Alkaline Smoothies Cookbook

Lose Weight with These Flavorful and Healthy Smoothies

Richard Ortega

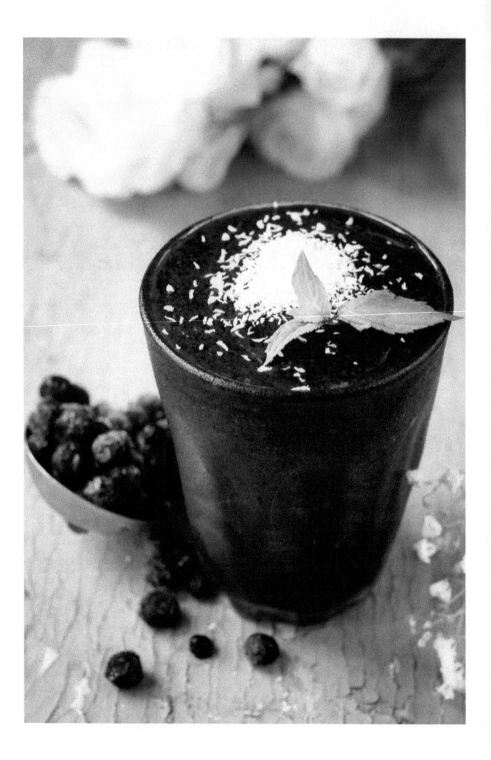

TABLE OF CONTENTS

Detox Berry Smoothie

Preparation Time: 10 minutes

Cooking Time: 0 minute

Servings: 2

Ingredients

- Spring water

- 1/4 avocado, pitted

- One medium burro banana

- One Seville orange

- Two cups of fresh lettuce

- One tablespoon of hemp seeds

- One cup of berries (blueberries or an aggregate of blueberries, strawberries, and raspberries)

Directions:

1. Add the spring water to your blender. Put the fruits and vegies right inside the blender.

2. Blend all ingredients till smooth.

Nutrition:

101 calories | 5.9g sugar | 14g protein

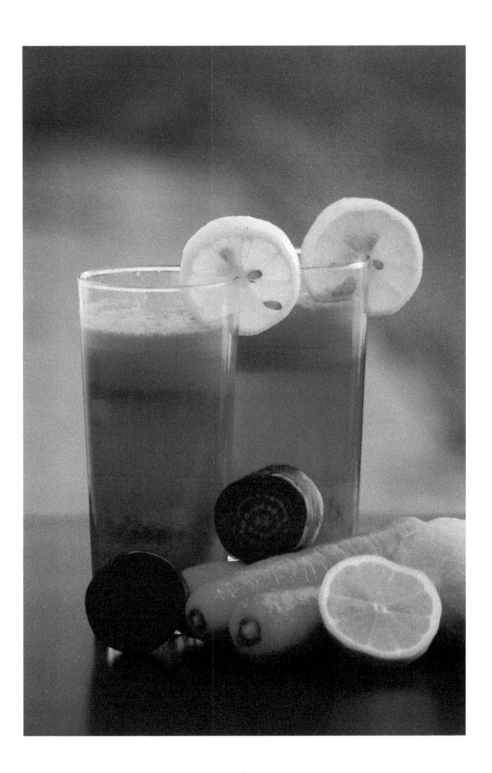

Papaya Detox Smoothie

Preparation Time: 10 minutes

Cooking Time: 0 minute

Servings: 2

Ingredients

- Two cups Papaya

- One tablespoon of papaya seeds

- Juice of a Lime

- One cup filtered water

Directions:

1. Chop the papaya into square portions and scoop out a tablespoon of clean and raw papaya seeds. Put all of the ingredients right into a high-speed blender for 1 minute until the whole thing is blended. Pour into a tumbler and enjoy this tasty drink your liver will love.

Nutrition:

94 calories | 2.5g sugar | 13g protein

Apple and Amaranth Detoxifying Smoothie

Preparation Time: 10 minutes

Cooking Time: 0 minute

Servings: 2

Ingredients

- 1/4 avocado

- 1 key lime

- 2 apples, chopped

- 2 cups of water

- 2 cups of Amaranth vegie

Directions:

1. Put all the ingredients collectively in a blender. Blend all the ingredients evenly

Nutrition:

105 calories | 3.9g sugar | 12g protein

Irish Sea Moss Smoothie

Preparation Time: 10 minutes

Cooking Time: 0 minute

Servings: 2

Ingredients

- 2 oz of whole, wild sea moss

- 2 cups of spring water

Directions:

1. To prepare Irish Sea Moss Smoothie, use two whole and wild sea moss. Carefully wash away any sand and debris. Soak it up to 24 hours in the spring water. This will increase the size of the sea moss. Do a final wash and chop up longer ones to safeguard your blender's blade. Add your soaked sea moss and two cups of spring water to blend in the blender. Put in a

jar and refrigerate. This smoothie can last for many weeks

Nutrition:

96 calories | 15g protein | 1.9g sugar

Peach Berry Smoothie

Preparation Time: 12 minutes

Cooking Time: 0 minute

Servings: 2

Ingredients

- Half cup of frozen peaches
- Half cup of frozen blueberries
- Half cup of frozen cherries
- Half cup of frozen strawberries
- One tablespoon of sea moss gel
- One tablespoon of hemp seeds
- One tablespoon of coconut water
- One tablespoon of agave

Directions:

1. Put all the above ingredients in a blender and blend for one minute. If the mixture is too thick, add extra ¼ cup of coconut water and blend for another 20 secs.

Nutrition:

106 calories | 16g protein | 9g sugar

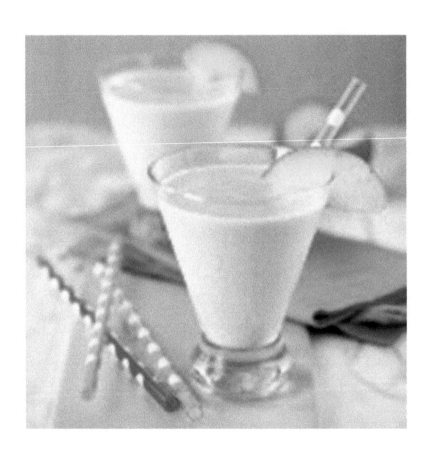

Cucumber Mixed Detox Smoothie

Preparation Time: 10 minutes

Cooking Time: 0 minute

Serving: 1

Ingredients

- Half cucumber, chopped

- One inch of ginger

- One pinch of pure sea salt

- Two grapefruits, squeezed

- Two lemons, squeezed

- One avocado, chopped

- Two cloves of sparkling garlic

- Half cup of filtered or spring water

- One pinch cayenne pepper

Directions:

1. Put all the ingredients into your blender and mix until thick and creamy.

2. Sip and experience this tasty nutritious smoothie!

Nutrition:

103 calories | 14g protein | 2g sugar

Avocado Mixed Smoothie

Preparation Time: 12 minutes

Cooking Time: 0 minute

Servings: 2

Ingredients

- One cup water
- One ounce of blueberries
- One pear, chopped
- 1/4 avocado, pitted
- 1/4 cup cooked quinoa

Directions:

1. Blend all ingredients in a high-speed blender and enjoy!

Nutrition:

99 calories | 15g protein | 2g sugar

Iron Power

Preparation Time: 15 minutes

Cooking Time: 0 minute

Servings: 2

Ingredients:

- 1 tsp. Bromide Plus Powder
- 1 tbsp Date sugar
- 2 handfuls Amaranth greens
- 1 cup Hemp seed milk,
- ½ cup Cooked quinoa
- 1 Fig
- 1 tbsp Raisins or currants
- ½ Large red apple

Directions:

1. Place the apple, raisins, fig, quinoa, milk, greens, sugar, and bromide plus powder into your blender.

Turn the blender on and let run until a creamy drink has been made.

Nutrition:

112 calories | 9g protein | 1g sugar

Sweet Sunrise

Preparation Time: 15 minutes

Cooking Time: 0 minute

Servings: 2

Ingredients:

- 1 cup Water

- 1 cup Mango

- ½ Burro banana

- 1 Seville orange

- 1 cup Raspberries

Directions:

1. Place the raspberries, orange, banana, mango, and water into your blender. Turn the blender on and let run until it forms a creamy drink.

Nutrition:

109 calories | 6g protein | 3.6g sugar

Coconut Lime

Preparation Time: 10 minutes

Cooking Time: 0 minute

Serving: 2

Ingredients:

- ½ cup Springwater
- 1 cup Ice
- 2 Key limes
- 1 cup Fresh coconut meat
- 1 Avocado
- Kale handful
- ½ cup Cucumber

Directions:

1. Place all the above ingredients into a blender and process until creamy and smooth.

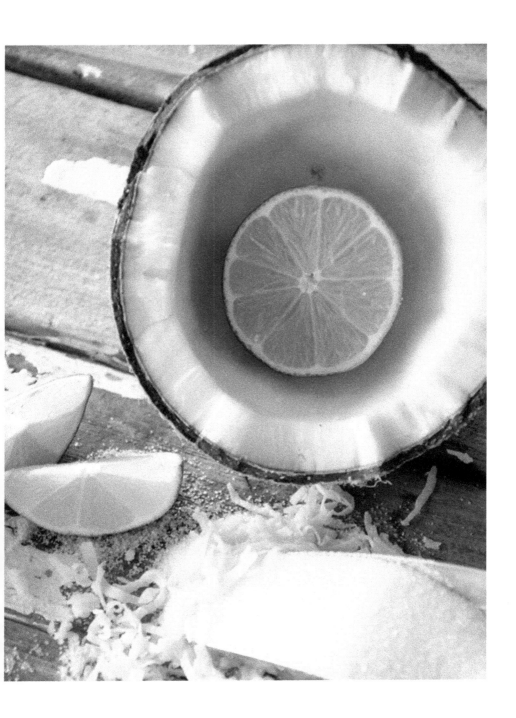

Wild Arugula Smoothie

Preparation Time: 10 minutes

Cooking Time: 0 minute

Serving: 1

Ingredients

- 2 medium bananas (chopped into bits)
- 1/2 cup of mango flesh pulp
- 1 cup of arugula (chopped into bits)
- 1/4 cup of blueberries
- 1 tablespoon of hemp seeds
- ½ tablespoon of bromide plus powder

Directions:

1. Pour all ingredients into a blender.
2. Blend for 30 seconds at a time until the mixture is smooth.

3. You may dilute with water to derive the desired thickness.

4. Serve in a cup and add some ice cubes or place in a refrigerator.

Nutrition:

103 calories | 4g sugar | 18g fiber

Turnip Berry Smoothie

Preparation Time: 10 minutes

Cooking Time: 0 minute

Serving: 1

Ingredients

- 1 cup of Turnip Greens (chopped into bits)
- ½ cup of water melon
- ½ cup of raspberries
- 1 tablespoon of sesame seeds

Directions:

1. Pour all ingredients into a blender.
2. Blend for 30 seconds at a time until the mixture is smooth.
3. You may dilute with water to derive the desired thickness.

4. Serve in a cup and add some ice cubes or place in a refrigerator.

Nutrition:

98 calories | 4.1g sugar | 19g protein

Veggie Avocado Smoothie

Preparation Time: 10 minutes

Cooking Time: 0 minute

Serving: 1

Ingredients

- 1 cup of lettuce
- 1 medium sized cucumber (chopped)
- 2 tablespoons of lime juice
- 1 tablespoon of ginger
- 1 medium sized avocado (peeled and mashed)
- ½ Apple (chopped into bits)
- 1 tablespoon of hempseeds

Directions:

1. Pour all ingredients into a blender.
2. Blend for 30 seconds at a time until the mixture is smooth.

3. You may dilute with water to derive the desired thickness.

4. Serve in a cup and add some ice cubes or place in a refrigerator.

Nutrition:

114 calories| 2g sugar | 11g fiber

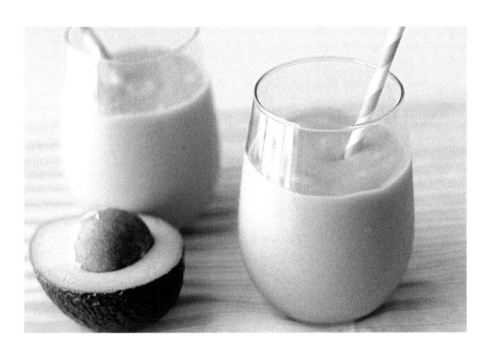

Amaranth Greens and Apple Smoothie

Preparation Time: 10 minutes

Cooking Time: 0 minute

Serving: 1

Ingredients

- 1 handful of amaranth green leaves
- 1 cup of blueberries and diced apples
- 2 tablespoons of lime juice
- 1 tablespoon of sea moss
- 1 tablespoon of hempseeds
- 1 cup of coconut milk

Directions:

1. Pour all ingredients into a blender.
2. Blend for 30 seconds at a time until the mixture is smooth.

3. You may dilute with water to derive the desired thickness.

4. Serve in a cup and add some ice cubes or place in a refrigerator.

Nutrition:

94 calories | 1g sugar | 10g protein

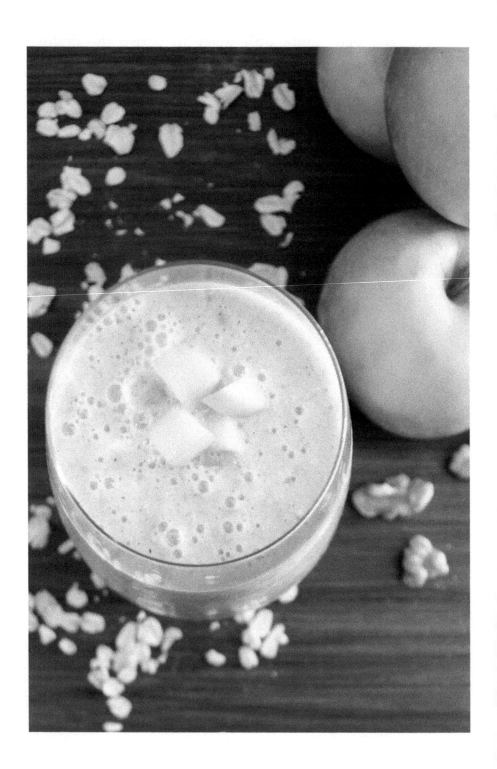

Double Berry Detox Smoothie

Preparation Time: 5 minutes

Cooking Time: 0 minute

Serving: 1

Ingredients

- ½ watermelon (chopped into bits)
- ½ cup each of strawberries and blueberries
- ¼ cup of orange juice with seeds
- 1 medium sized banana
- 2 cups of lettuce
- 1 peach (chopped into bits)

Directions:

1. Pour all ingredients into a blender.
2. Blend for 30 seconds at a time until the mixture is smooth.

3. You may dilute with water to derive the desired thickness.

4. Serve in a cup and add some ice cubes or place in a refrigerator.

Nutrition:

111 calories | 5g fat | 3g sugar

Kale Citrus Berry Detox Smoothie

Preparation Time: 10 minutes

Cooking Time: 0 minute

Serving: 1

Ingredients

- 1 medium sized banana (chopped into bits)
- ½ cup of strawberries
- 1 cup of Arugula (chopped into bits)
- 1 tablespoon of lime juice
- ¼ cup of orange juice with seeds
- 1 cup of coconut water
- ½ tablespoon of sea moss

Directions:

1. Pour all ingredients into a blender.

2. Blend for 30 seconds at a time until the mixture is smooth.

3. You may dilute with water to derive the desired thickness.

4. Serve in a cup and add some ice cubes or place in a refrigerator.

Nutrition:

113 calories | 6g fiber | 1g sugar

Banana Soursop Berry Toxin Flush Smoothie

Preparation Time: 15 minutes

Cooking Time: 0 minute

Serving: 1

Ingredients

- 2 medium sized bananas (chopped into bits)
- ½ cup of strawberry or raspberry
- 1 cup of soursop pulp
- 1 cup each of Kale and Lettuce (chopped into bits)
- ½ tablespoon of sea moss

Directions:

1. Pour all ingredients into a blender.
2. Blend for 30 seconds at a time until the mixture is smooth.

3. You may dilute with water to derive the desired thickness.

4. Serve in a cup and add some ice cubes or place in a refrigerator.

Nutrition:

105 calories | 8g fiber | 4g sugar

Green Toxin Flusher Smoothie

Preparation Time: 10 minutes

Cooking Time: 0 minute

Serving: 1

Ingredients

- 2 medium sized bananas (chopped into bits)
- 1 cup of diced cucumber
- 1 cup each of Kale and Lettuce (chopped into bits)
- 1/4 cup of lime juice
- ½ tablespoon of sea moss
- 1 teaspoon of date sugar

Direction:

1. Pour all ingredients into a blender.
2. Blend for 30 seconds at a time until the mixture is smooth.

3. You may dilute with water to derive the desired thickness.

4. Serve in a cup and add some ice cubes or place in a refrigerator.

Nutrition:

99 calories | 7g fiber | 2g sugar

Kale Smoothie

Preparation Time: 10 minutes

Cooking Time: 0 minute

Servings: 1

Ingredients

- 2 medium apples (chopped into bits)
- 1/2 cup of diced cucumber
- 1 cup of Kale (chopped into bits)
- 1/4 cup of coconut milk
- ½ tablespoon of sea moss

Directions:

1. Pour all ingredients into a blender.
2. Blend for 30 seconds at a time until the mixture is smooth.
3. You may dilute with water to derive the desired thickness.

4. Serve in a cup and add some ice cubes or place in a refrigerator.

Nutrition:

89 calories | 8g protein | 1g sugar

Alkaline Raspberry Smoothie

Preparation Time: 10 minutes

Cooking Time: 0 minute

Serving: 1

Ingredients

- 2 cups of raspberries

- 1/4 cup of coconut water

- ¼ cup of spinach leaves (chopped)

- ½ tablespoon of hempseeds and bromide plus powder

- 4 dates (soaked in water)

Directions:

1. Pour all ingredients into a blender.

2. Blend for 30 seconds at a time until the mixture is smooth.

3. You may dilute with water to derive the desired thickness.

4. Serve in a cup and add some ice cubes or place in a refrigerator.

Nutrition:

111 calories | 5g fiber | 1g sugar

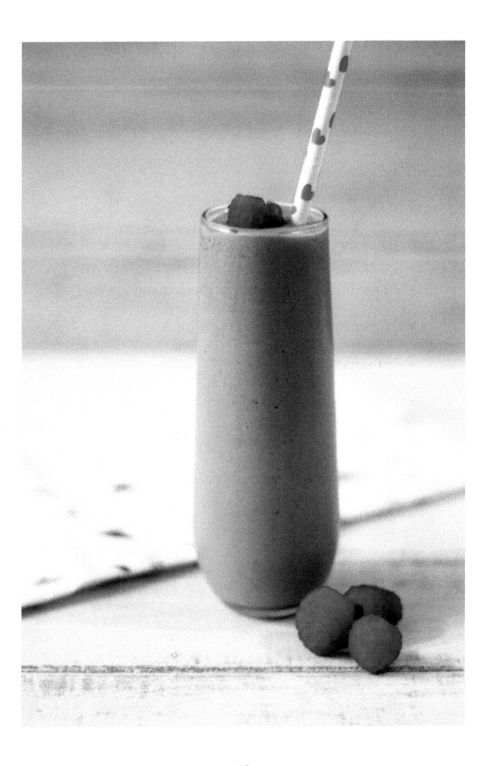

Creamy Avocado Smoothie

Preparation Time: 10 minutes

Cooking Time: 0 minute

Serving: 1

Ingredients

- 3 medium sized avocados (peeled and mashed)
- 1/2 cucumber (chopped into bits)
- 1 teaspoon of oregano
- 3 teaspoons of orange juice
- 1/2 cup of Kale leaves (chopped)
- 1 tablespoon of sea moss powder
- 2 dates (soaked in water)

Directions:

1. Pour all ingredients into a blender.
2. Blend for 30 seconds at a time until the mixture is smooth.

3. You may dilute with water to derive the desired thickness.

4. Serve in a cup and add some ice cubes or place in a refrigerator.

Nutrition:

100 calories | 1g sugar | 5g fats

Veggie Detox Smoothie

Preparation Time: 10 minutes

Cooking Time: 0 minute

Serving: 1

Ingredients

- ¼ cup of coconut milk
- 1 teaspoon of olive oil
- 1 cup of spinach juice
- 1 teaspoon of agave syrup
- 1/2 cup of lettuce (chopped)
- ½ red onion (diced)
- ½ teaspoon of cayenne

Directions:

1. Pour all ingredients into a blender.
2. Blend for 30 seconds at a time until the mixture is smooth.

3. You may dilute with water to derive the desired thickness.

4. Serve in a cup and add some ice cubes or place in a refrigerator.

Nutrition:

108 calories | 4g fats | 2g sugar

Kale Spinach Detoxifying Smoothie

Preparation Time: 10 minutes

Cooking Time: 0 minute

Serving: 1

Ingredients

- 1/2 cup of spinach juice
- 2 tablespoons of lime juice
- 1 teaspoon of agave syrup
- 1 cup of Kale leaves (chopped)
- ½ apple (chopped into bits)
- ½ teaspoon of cayenne and bromide plus powder

Directions:

1. Pour all ingredients into a blender.
2. Blend for 30 seconds at a time until the mixture is smooth.

3. You may dilute with water to derive the desired thickness.

4. Serve in a cup and add some ice cubes or place in a refrigerator.

Nutrition:

79 calories | 5g fats | 1g sugar

Peachy Spinach Smoothie

Preparation Time: 10 minutes

Cooking Time: 0 minute

Serving: 1

Ingredients

- 1/2 cup of spinach juice
- 2 tablespoons of lime juice
- 1 medium sized banana
- 1 cup of lettuce (chopped)
- ½ cup of peach
- ½ cucumber (chopped into bits)
- ½ teaspoon of cayenne and bromide plus powder

Directions:

1. Pour all ingredients into a blender.
2. Blend for 30 seconds at a time until the mixture is smooth.

3. You may dilute with water to derive the desired thickness.

4. Serve in a cup and add some ice cubes or place in a refrigerator.

Nutrition:

115 calories | 6g fiber | 0.9g sugar

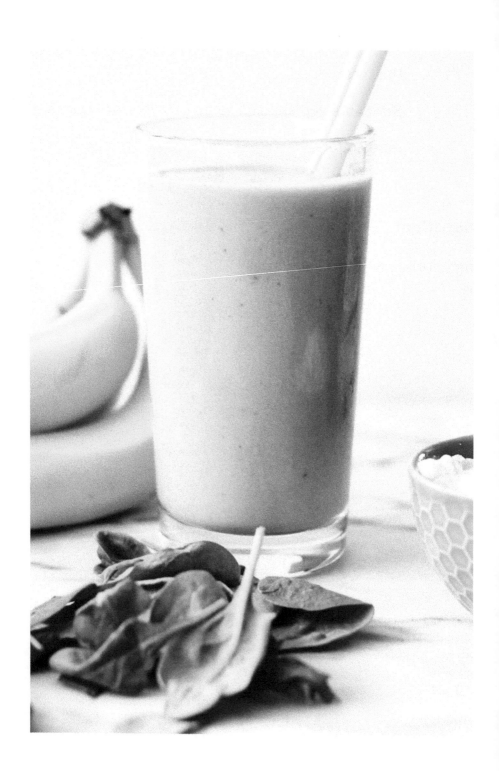

Fruity Refreshing Smoothie

Preparation Time: 10 minutes

Cooking Time: 0 minute

Serving: 1

Ingredients

- 3 tablespoons of lime juice
- 2 medium sized Apple (chopped into bits)
- 2 tablespoons of agave syrup
- 3 cucumbers (medium sized – chopped into bits)
- 3 cups of water melon (chopped into bits)
- 1 tablespoon of mint leaves

Directions:

1. Put all melon, cucumber and apple in a blender and blend for 30 seconds at a time. Squeeze and sieve the juice from the ensuing mixture and pour the juice into a bowl.

2. Add the lime juice and agave syrup to the juice until you obtain the desired sweetness. You may also add water to lighten the thickness of the juice.

3. Sprinkle some mint leaves on the Drink and add some ice cubes.

Nutrition:

109 calories | 9g fiber | 4g sugar | 19g protein

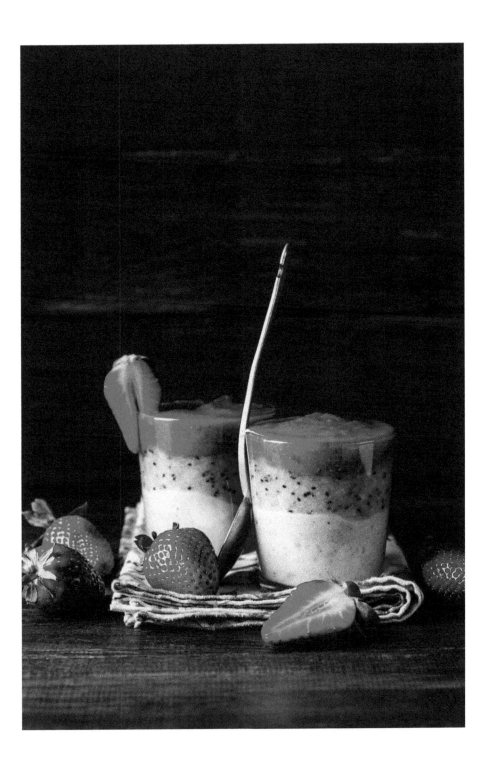

Veggie-full Smoothie

Preparation Time: 10 minutes

Cooking Time: 0 minute

Servings: 2

Ingredients:

- 1 pear

- ¼ avocado

- ½ cucumber

- 1 watercress

- 1 lettuce

- ½ cup spring water

- Date sugar to taste

Directions:

1. Blend all ingredients until smooth.

Nutrition:

98 calories | 15g fiber | 9g fats

"Apple Pie" Smoothie

Preparation Time: 10 minutes

Cooking Time: 0 minute

Serving: 1

Ingredients:

- ½ large apples
- 2 figs
- Small handful of walnuts
- 1 cup ginger tea
- 1 tbsp date sugar
- 1 tsp bromide Plus Powder

Directions:

1. Prepare the ginger tea and let it to cool. Blend the rest of the ingredients.

Nutrition:

109 calories | 1g sugar | 5g fiber

Sea Moss Berry

Preparation Time: 10 minutes

Cooking Time: 0 minute

Serving: 2

Ingredients

- 1 large handful greens
- ½ cup of mixed berries
- 1/2 banana (frozen)
- 1 freshly squeezed lime
- 1 tbsp sea moss
- 1 cup coconut water

Directions:

1. Blend all the ingredients until smooth.

Nutrition:

99 calories | 8g protein | 2g sugar

Berry Greens

Preparation Time: 15 minutes

Cooking Time: 0 minute

Servings: 2

Ingredients:

- 1 handful greens

- 1 cup raspberries (frozen)

- 2 tbsp lime juice

- 1 cup coconut milk

- 1 tbsp. sea moss

Directions:

1. Blend all the ingredients until smooth.

Nutrition:

98 calories | 3g sugar | 11g protein

Apple Berry

Preparation Time: 10 minutes

Cooking Time: 0 minute

Servings: 2

Ingredients:

- 1 cup mixed berry

- 1 large apple

- 2 cups greens

- 1 cup water

Directions

1. Blend all the ingredients until smooth.

Nutrition:

110 calories| 9g fiber | 17g protein

Banana Berry Veggie

Preparation Time: 15 minutes

Cooking Time: 0 minute

Servings: 2

Ingredients:

- 1 banana
- 1 cup frozen strawberry
- 1 cup kale
- 1 cup ice

Directions:

1. Blend all the ingredients until smooth.

Nutrition:

96 calories | 9g fiber | 12g protein

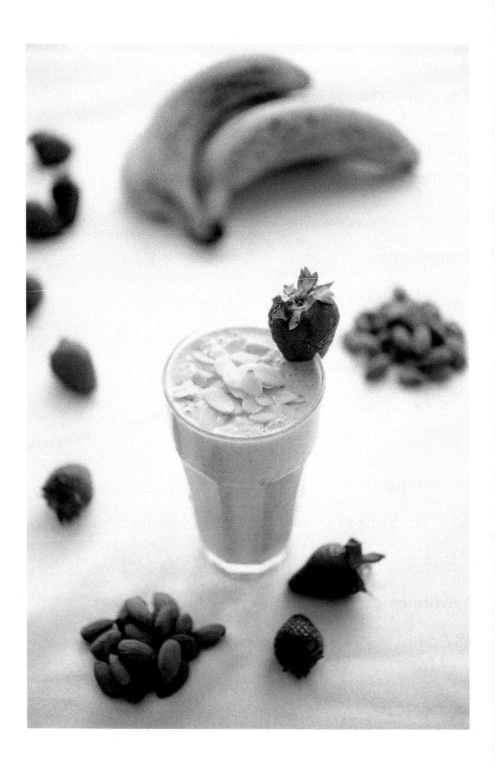

Leafy Greens

Preparation Time: 10 minutes

Cooking Time: 0 minute

Serving: 1

Ingredients:

- 1 handful greens
- 1/2 lime
- 1-inch fresh ginger
- 1/2 cucumber
- 1 cup coconut water
- 1 date

Directions:

1. Blend all the ingredients until smooth.

Nutrition:

91 calories | 5g fiber | 1g sugar

Fruity Flax

Preparation Time: 10 minutes

Cooking time: 0 minute

Serving: 1

Ingredients:

- 2 cups greens
- ½ cup blueberry
- 1 frozen banana
- 1 tbsp. flaxseeds
- 1 cup water

Directions:

1. Blend all the ingredients until smooth.

Nutrition:

105 calories | 2g sugar | 7g fiber

Apple Juice Mix

Preparation Time: 5 minutes

Cooking Time: 0 minute

Serving: 2

Ingredients:

- 1 1/2 cup apple juice
- 2 cups steamed kale
- 1 apple
- 1/2 avocado

Directions:

1. Blend all the ingredients until smooth.

Nutrition:

93 calories | 14g protein | 2g sugar

Banana Coconut

Preparation Time: 10 minutes

Cooking Time: 0 minute

Servings: 2

Ingredients:

- 1 banana
- 1 pear
- 1 cup coconut water
- 2 cups kale

Directions

1. Blend all the ingredients until smooth.

Nutrition:

91 calories | 2g sugar | 14g protein

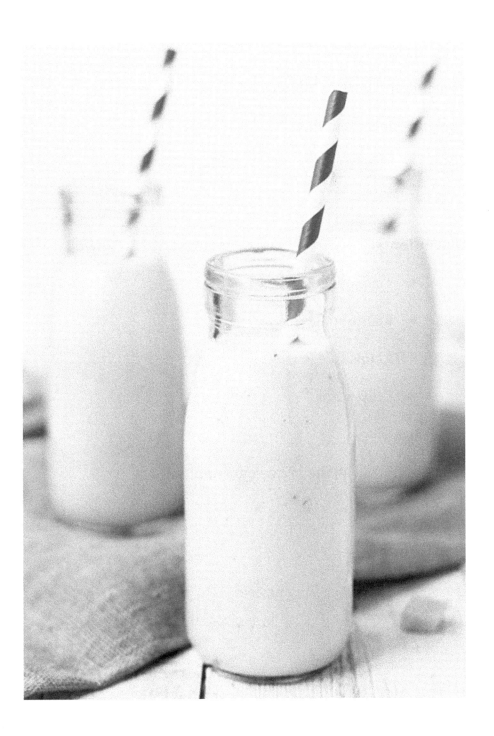

Berry Kale Delight

Preparation Time: 10 minutes

Cooking Time: 0 minute

Serving: 1

Ingredients:

- 1 cup mixed berries
- 1 large apple
- 2 cups kale
- 1 cup water

Directions

1. Blend all the ingredients until smooth.

Nutrition:

110 calories | 5g fiber | 14g protein

Lime Banana Smoothie

Preparation Time: 15 minutes

Cooking Time: 0 minute

Serving: 2

Ingredients

- 1/2 burro banana
- 1 cup Romaine lettuce
- 2 – 3 tbsp key lime juice
- 1/2 cup ginger tea
- 1/4 cup blueberries
- 1/2 cup soft jelly coconut water

Directions:

1. Prepare the ginger tea and let it cool. Blend all the ingredients until smooth.

Nutrition:

112 calories | 2g sugar | 19g protein

Tea Delight Smoothie

Preparation Time: 10 minutes

Cooking Time: 0 minute

Serving: 2

Ingredients:

- 1 burro banana
- 1/4 cup prepared Alkaline's Nerve/Stress Relief Herbal Tea
- 1/2 cup homemade walnut milk
- 1 tbsp date sugar

Directions:

1. Prepare the tea and let it cool. Blend all the ingredients until smooth.

Nutrition:

98 calories | 1g sugar | 10g fiber

Iron Apple Smoothie

Preparation Time: 10 minutes

Cooking Time: 0 minute

Servings: 2

Ingredients

- ½ large apple
- 1 tbsp raisins
- 1 fig
- ½ cup cooked quinoa
- 1 cup homemade seed milk
- 2 handfuls amaranth greens
- 1 tbsp date sugar
- 1 tsp. Bromide Plus Powder

Directions:

1. Blend all the ingredients until smooth.

Nutrition:

103 calories | 2g fats | 17g protein

Green Detox Smoothie

Preparation Time: 15 minutes

Cooking Time: 0 minute

Serving: 1

Ingredients

- ½ burro banana
- 1 cup lettuce
- 2 – 3 tbsp key lime juice
- 1/2 cup ginger tea
- 1/4 cup blueberries
- 1/2 cup soft jelly coconut water

Directions:

1. Prepare the tea and let it cool. Blend all the ingredients until smooth.

Nutrition:

104 calories | 9g fiber | 1g sugar

Watercress Smoothie

Preparation Time: 5 minutes

Cooking Time: 0 minute

Serving 2

Ingredients

- 2 cups spring water
- 1 large bunch of dandelion greens, fresh
- ¼ cup key lime juice
- 1 cup of watercress, fresh
- 3 baby bananas, peeled
- ½ cup fresh blueberries
- 1-inch piece of ginger, fresh
- 6 Medjool dates, pitted
- 1 tablespoon burdock root powder

Directions:

1. Take a high-powered blender, switch it on, and then place all the ingredients inside, in order.

2. Cover the blender with its lid and then pulse at high speed for 1 minute.

Nutrition:

102 calories | 2g sugar | 11g fiber

Three Berry Smoothie

Preparation Time: 15 minutes

Cooking Time: 0 minute

Serving: 1

Ingredients

- 1 cup spring water
- 1 cup fresh whole strawberries
- 2 small bananas
- 1 cup fresh whole raspberries
- 2 tablespoons agave syrup
- 1 cup fresh whole blueberries

Directions:

1. Take a high-powered blender, switch it on, and then place all the ingredients inside, in order.
2. Cover the blender with its lid and then pulse at high speed for 1 minute.

Nutrition:

98 calories | 5g fiber | 10g protein

Watermelon Lime Smoothie

Preparation Time: 15 minutes

Cooking Time: 0 minute

Serving: 1

Ingredients

- 4 cups watermelon, deseeded, cubed
- 4 key limes, juiced
- 4 cucumbers, deseeded, sliced

Directions:

1. Take a high-powered blender, switch it on, and then place all the ingredients inside, in order.
2. Cover the blender with its lid and then pulse at high speed for 1 minute.

Nutrition:

102 calories | 2g sugar | 5g fiber

Lettuce Citrus Smoothie

Preparation Time: 5 minutes

Cooking Time: 0 minute

Servings: 2

Ingredients

- 1 cup coconut water
- 1 cup lettuce leaves, fresh
- 1 key lime, juiced
- 1 Seville orange, peeled
- 1 tablespoon bromide plus powder
- ½ of a medium avocado, pitted

Directions:

1. Take a high-powered blender, switch it on, and then place all the ingredients inside, in order.

2. Cover the blender with its lid and then pulse at high speed for 1 minute.

Nutrition:

97 calories | 4g fats | 11g fiber

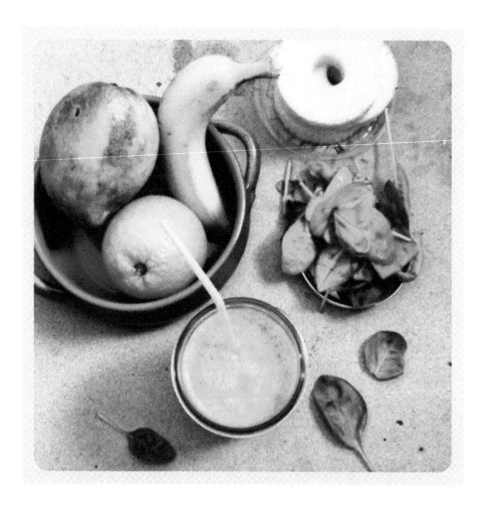

Fruity Quinoa Smoothie

Preparation Time: 15 minutes

Cooking Time: 0 minute

Serving: 1

Ingredients

- 2 cups spring water
- ½ of avocado, pitted
- 2 fresh pears, chopped
- ½ cup cooked quinoa
- ¼ cup fresh whole blueberries

Directions:

1. Take a high-powered blender, switch it on, and then place all the ingredients inside, in order.

2. Cover the blender with its lid and then pulse at high speed for 1 minute.

Nutrition:

98 calories | 14g protein | 7g fiber

Mango Banana Smoothie

Preparation Time: 15 minutes

Cooking Time: 0 minute

Servings: 1

Ingredients

- 1 cup spring water

- 2 cups greens

- ½ of banana, peeled

- 1 fresh mango, peeled, destoned, sliced

Directions:

1. Take a high-powered blender, switch it on, and then place all the ingredients inside, in order.

2. Cover the blender with its lid and then pulse at high speed for 1 minute.

Nutrition:

95 calories | 6g fiber | 10g protein

Toxin Flush Smoothie

Preparation Time: 15 minutes

Cooking Time: 0 minute

Serving: 1

Ingredients:

- A key lime
- A cucumber
- Cubed, seeded watermelon, 1 c

Direction:

1. Wash and dice the cucumber. Add the watermelon and cucumber to the blender and mix until combined. You shouldn't need to add extra water since both the watermelon and cucumber are mainly water.

2. Slice the lime in half and squeeze the juice into your smoothie. Enjoy.

Nutrition:

111 calories | 4g fiber | 1g sugar

Berry Peach Smoothie

Preparation Time: 5 minutes

Cooking Time: 5 minutes

Serves: 2

Ingredients

- 1 cup coconut water
- 1 tbsp. hemp seeds
- 1 tbsp. agave
- 1/2 cup strawberries
- 1/2 cup blueberries
- 1/2 cup cherries
- 1/2 cup peaches

Directions:

1. Place all the ingredients into a blender then blend until they become smooth and creamy. Serve.

Nutrition:

98 calories | 6g fiber | 2g sugar

Veggie Avocado Smoothie

Preparation Time: 5 minutes

Cooking Time: 5 minutes

Serving: 3

Ingredients

- 1 cup water

- 1/2 peeled Seville orange

- 1 avocado

- 1 peeled cucumber

- 1 cup kale

- 1 cup ice cubes

Directions:

1. Place all the ingredients into a blender then process until they are smooth and creamy. Serve and enjoy.

Nutrition:

104 calories | 4g fiber | 9g protein

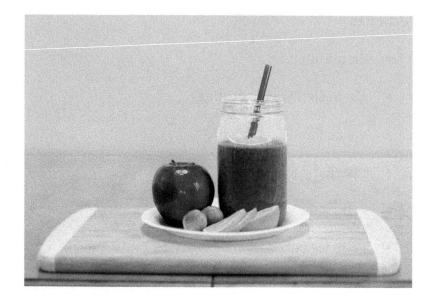

Apple Blueberry Smoothie

Preparation Time: 15 minutes

Cooking Time: 0 minute

Serving: 1

Ingredients:

- 1/2 apple
- 1 Date
- 1/2 cup blueberries
- 1/2 cup sparkling callaloo
- 1 tbsp. hemp seeds
- 1 tbsp. sesame seeds
- 2 cups sparkling soft-jelly coconut water
- 1/2 tbsp. bromide plus powder

Directions:

1. Mix all the ingredients in a high-speed blender. Serve and enjoy!

Nutrition:

98 calories | 3g sugar | 17g protein

30 DAY MEAL PLAN

Day	Breakfast	Main Dishes	Snacks
1	Blackberry Pie	Kamut Burger	Avocado Basil Pasta
2	Blueberry Spelt Breakfast Muffins	Veggie Burgers	Rice and Spinach Balls
3	Alkaline Blueberry Breakfast Cake	Falafel with Tzatziki Sauce	Flatbread
4	Teff Sausages	Veggie Kabobs	Enoki Mushroom Pasta
5	Alkaline Breakfast Biscuits	Mushroom Curry	Walnut Kale Pasta
6	Zucchini Bacon	Veggies Casserole	Tomato Pasta
7	Alkaline Spelt Bread	Sweet and Spicy Chickpeas	Zucchini Tomato Pasta
8	Alkaline Crustless Quiche	Chickpea and Veggies Stew	Zucchini Bacon
9	Alkaline's Home Fries Hash Browns	Alkaline Pizza Crust	Alkaline Sausage Links
10	Alkaline Blueberry and Strawberry Muffins	Vegan Alkaline Ribs	Garlicky Broccoli
11	Teff Breakfast Porridge	Grilled Zucchini Hummus Wrap	Sautéed Kale
12	Alkaline Sausage Links	Veggie Fajitas Tacos	Parsley Mushrooms
13	Breakfast Blueberry Bars	Chickpea Mashed Potatoes	Speltbread
14	Alkaline Veggie Omelet	Wild Rice and Black Lentil Bowl	Tortillas
15	Butternut Squash	Cauliflower	Tortilla Chips

	Hash Browns	Alfredo Pasta	
16	Blueberry Spelt Flat Cakes	Zucchini Noodles with Avocado Sauce	Onion Rings
17	Blueberry Pie	Chinese Cucumber Salad Magnifico	Basil and Olive Pizza
18	Blueberry Spelt Breakfast Muffins	Artichoke Sauce Ala Quinoa Pasta	Tomato Spelt Pasta
19	Alkaline Blueberry Breakfast Cake	Beautifully Curried Eggplant	Tropical Mushrooms
20	Teff Sausages	Coconut Milk and Glazing Stir Fried Tofu	Shortbread Cookies
21	Alkaline Breakfast Biscuits	Culturally Diverse Pumpkin Potato Patties	Coconut Cookies
22	Zucchini Bacon	Italian Leek Fry	Blueberry Mousse
23	Alkaline Spelt Bread	Almond and Celery Mix of Delight	Almond Pulp Cookies
24	Alkaline Crustless Quiche	Spicy Tofu Burger	Toasted Trail Mix
25	Alkaline's Home Fries Hash Browns	Special Pasta Ala Pepper and Tomato Sauce	Chickpea Avocado Cups
26	Alkaline Blueberry and Strawberry Muffins	Southern Amazing Salad	Toasty Quinoa
27	Teff Breakfast Porridge	Pad Thai	Tropical Pancakes
28	Alkaline Sausage Links	Yellow Squash and Bell Pepper Bake	Quinoa Grout
29	Breakfast Blueberry Bars	Bell Peppers and Tomato Casserole	Squash Hash

| 30 | Alkaline Veggie Omelet | Nori-Burritos | Blackberry Pie |

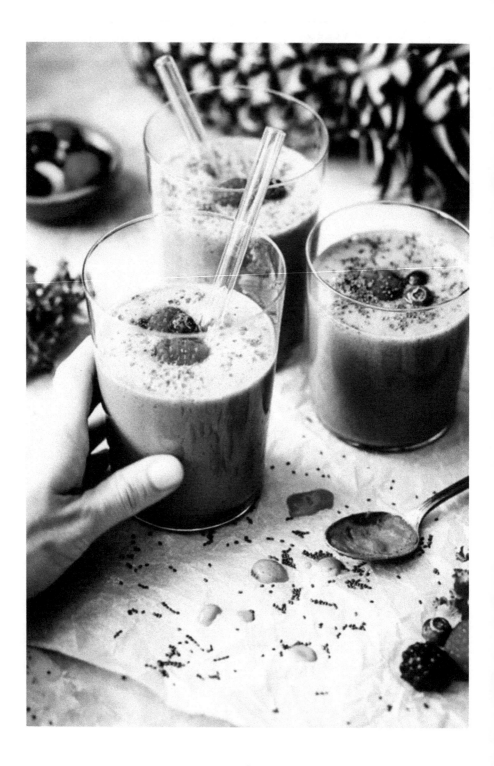

Lightning Source UK Ltd.
Milton Keynes UK
UKHW020803160621
385600UK00005B/25